Active Again

by
HEATHER STOTT

clearing
my chronic fatigue
and coeliac minefield

© Heather Stott

First published February 2002

ISBN 0-9542409-0-1

Published by
Tulip Press
26 Station Road
South Cave
Brough
East Yorkshire HU15 2AA
United Kingdom

e-mail address
active@tulippress.freeserve.co.uk

web site
www.chronicfatiguesyndrome.co.uk

Printed by Central Print Services,
The University of Hull

INTRODUCTION

Disillusion, frustration and fury motivated me to write this account of the course of my life over the past eight and a half years. With better, open minded, medical diagnosis and treatment I believe that this phase of my life would not have been wasted.

I know that I am not alone in having suffered a myriad of unexplained symptoms. If this chronicle of my experiences helps one other person to get to the cause of their ill-health then writing this will have been worthwhile.

I am fifty seven years old and was afflicted by a set of debilitating symptoms when I was forty eight. It has taken a very long time to sort out all my problems. The complications have been such that I have likened it to clearing a pathway through a minefield. However I was determined, even at my lowest ebb, that I was not going to accept permanent ill health.

This is not a tale of how I tried complementary or alternative therapies, I have only been prepared to accept advice and treatment from qualified doctors, although some of the treatments are what many members of the medical profession would regard as controversial. Following these treatments for the last three years there has been a gradual and continuing improvement in my health until I am now back to my old self.

What were my symptoms?

Originally I was struck down by extreme weakness in my thigh muscles which then spread to several of my other muscles. Also I had severe, frequently excruciating, muscle pains and muscle twitchings all over the body, particularly in the major muscles of the legs and arms. In the early period I suffered muscle squirmings which looked as if I had a large number of worms crawling under the surface of the skin.

Later as the years passed I noticed my hair was falling out, also my eyebrows and eyelashes. I completely lost my sense of taste and smell and became extremely sensitive to noise and cold, and later to the computer, microwave and telephone. My brain wouldn't function, I couldn't concentrate. In addition I developed aches and pains in my fingers, knees and knuckles.

At times I have put on as much as two stones in weight as a result of fluid retention. I have also experienced bowel disturbances, loss of balance, different sorts of rashes, sore tongue, dry prickly eyes, tinnitus, earache, shocks on the scalp and arms, allergies, bloating, dry lips, eczema, a persistent dry cough, numbness and tingling, diabetes, hypoglycaemia, an abnormal heart rhythm and candida. Frequently all of them at the same time.

With whom am I disillusioned?

Narrow minded members of the medical profession who gave me the impression that they were not really applying their minds to what I said, consequently I felt as if I had been imprisoned when innocent.

I have been prodded, poked and patronised by experts. Some problems have been isolated, some problems treated and, I suppose not surprisingly, some problems created by the transient attention of one doctor or another, but for a long period of time the underlying symptoms remained as debilitating as ever.

It is not easy to continue to search for the cause of ill-health when the doctors' attitudes are grinding you down but you must have determination.

Why was I frustrated?

Until I was struck down I had led an active outdoor life. Then for six of the past eight years in one of my better periods I might manage to walk a few hundred yards, but afterwards I would need prolonged bed rest to recover.

Watching the buds and leaves breaking into colour on the shrubs and trees year after year made me realize how the time was passing.

However pleasant or attractive the surroundings all I wanted was to be back to normal health.

Why am I furious?

Like thousands of other sufferers of a myriad of unexplained symptoms I did not consider and still do not consider that I have had all the help and support that was needed from the caring professions. Even when advice or treatment was proffered the lack of adequate explanation or communication left me confused and worried, and exacerbated the situation.

The result of this was to leave me feeling a nuisance.

The arrogance of some members of the medical professions is unbelievable and is not conducive to patient calmness and well-being. It only serves to increase the stress levels thereby making the symptoms worse, and instilling a doctor phobia of the most destructive type whereby the patient is reluctant not only to return to that doctor but also reluctant to risk potential exposure to the same experience with another doctor.

The lack of continuous and sympathetic help from the medical professions served to push me, like so many others, to look outside the N.H.S. for treatment.

It has been a long hard and very expensive journey. Having to spend over fourteen thousand pounds should not have been necessary.

This is my story. I am not a doctor and I am not recommending any particular type of treatment for any other sufferer, but I hope that some of the information may help to point you in the right direction.

CHAPTER 1

One day in August 1993 when I was walking up the hill on my way home from the shops I had a peculiar feeling in my right thigh muscle. It was a sensation of extreme weakness, as if there was no muscle there, something I had never experienced before.

As this sensation in my muscle became stronger my leg went weaker and weaker until I could hardly bear any weight on it. I reached home with great difficulty, dragging the leg along.

For the next four days I was not very well at all. Pains and severe twitching developed in a lot of muscles throughout my body and I was weak with no energy.

By this time I thought that I had probably just got a bug, but I did not have a temperature or cough or cold and was reluctant to go to the doctor thinking that it would soon pass.

I love walking and had walked ten miles a couple of days before feeling ill so I thought that there could not be much wrong with me. My husband, Colin, and I had been to Scarborough, which is about fifty miles from our home, and walked seven miles from the south side along the front to the north side and back. The day before that I had played a full round of golf, which involved a walk of about three miles.

On the fifth day, thinking I would be well enough, I drove ten miles to the nearest town to do some shopping. When I was in WH Smiths my legs suddenly went very weak and I had to ask for assistance. The staff in the shop were very helpful and telephoned Colin to come to take me home, leaving my car to be recovered later.

Although I did not realize it at the time this was my first lesson in the impact that this illness, whatever it was, was going to have on my independence and my self-confidence.

The next day I decided that I had better visit the doctor. He took some blood and said to come back in a week for the results.

A couple of days after this we began to worry as I was going downhill rapidly and could hardly walk from room to room. We decided that I had better pay the doctor another visit. As it was my doctor's day off I saw another doctor. Without the laboratory results the best this doctor could suggest was to stop drinking coffee and to take anti-inflammatory pills.

Two days later Colin was working fifty miles away and after a morning in bed I thought I would be able to get up to get myself some lunch. I was sadly mistaken. I found my legs would not support me at all and was very frightened.

Using the telephone by the bed I managed to call a friend to ask her if she would come and make me a drink so that I could take some pills. I felt bad about this as she was very busy preparing for her silver wedding party the next day. She and her husband rushed round but could not get in as the door was locked. I had to crawl on my hands and knees from my bed to the front door, which I found very difficult because of my weakness. Fortunately we live in a bungalow. My friends helped me back to bed and rang the doctor.

My G.P. arrived quickly and having examined me decided it would be better if I went into the local infirmary. Within an hour or so I was in hospital, having rung Colin while waiting for the ambulance.

I was superficially examined by a junior doctor and I showed her the involuntary movement in my thigh muscles. I can only describe this as looking as if there were hundreds of maggots crawling just below the surface of the skin. It was a revolting sensation.

As it was a Friday preceding a bank holiday weekend all departments would be closed for routine diagnostic testing until the following Tuesday. No way did I want to stay in hospital if nothing was going to be done so the next morning I persuaded the doctor to let me go home until tests could be arranged.

When my daughter came to visit me I explained that I could go home. She found a wheelchair so that she could take me to the car to bring me home. Even after only one night in hospital it was lovely to be back in my own surroundings for the weekend so I tried to relax as best I could, but this was not easy and I wasn't very successful.

Lying in bed at night all sorts of dreadful thoughts about what could be wrong with me were whizzing around my brain and the constant pain meant that sleep did not come easily. I hoped that my symptoms would disappear over the next couple of days so that I would not have to return to the ward.

There was no change by Tuesday morning so off I went, in trepidation, back to the hospital. I was very anxious.

My anxiety was not helped by the fact that it was a mixed sex neurological ward. I soon discovered that the men snored badly and some men shouted a lot in the night. One man in particular was anti-women and shouted obscenities at the nurses throughout the day and night. He abused the nurses very badly.

Some patients chatted to me about their illnesses in great detail. In the next bed was a woman in her early forties who had suffered a stroke. A few days later she had a brain operation to remove a blood clot. It gave me the creeps to hear everybody's tales of their brain tumours and strokes, and it made me wonder what on earth might be causing my muscular problems.

Throughout the next week in hospital I had a brain and neck scan, blood tests, and a test where wires were attached to my head, fingers and toes to see if the electrical impulses from my brain were reaching my extremities. I likened this latter experience to being in an electric chair, although these tests were not painful.

All the tests were clear. This was a relief, but on the other hand we were no nearer to finding the cause of my illness.

During this week I suffered the first of many very upsetting experiences because of lack of understanding by all levels of the medical profession.

I had been managing to shuffle very slowly to the toilet when necessary, but on one occasion my legs became so weak that I had to be taken back to my bed in a wheelchair. A nurse told me not to try to walk there again but to buzz for a wheelchair.

Later the same day during visiting time when all the beds had visitors sitting around them I needed to go to the toilet. I pressed the buzzer. A different nurse came and told me that I did not need a wheelchair, I could walk. Being too weak to argue I tried to do as I was told. Putting her arm through mine the nurse started to walk far faster than I could manage half dragging me along. After a few paces I was on the point of collapse.

The visitors and patients, some in tears at what they were seeing, decided that enough was enough and one of them thrust a chair under me as I collapsed. The nurse begrudgingly produced a wheelchair and took me to the toilet, telling me to pull the call cord when I was ready to return to my bed. This I did several times but nobody came for what seemed a very long time.

I decided this was her way of punishing me for being difficult.

When I was back in bed I was exhausted. The patient in the bed opposite came across to sympathise and explained that she had been to tell the sister what had happened, consequently sister came to talk to me to obtain my version of events. I told her that I did not want that nurse to come near me again.

This sort of experience only served to increase my anxiety. Unfortunately this was only the first of several very unpleasant, unnecessary incidents.

By Friday I could not wait to go home again for the weekend. Monday morning arrived and I really did not want to return to the ward but steeled myself because I was scheduled to have another electrical test. This test was unpleasant as needles were inserted into my leg muscles and an electric current passed between the needles and a machine. This test was also negative.

The consultant decided on the basis of all the results that I was suffering from transient post-viral myalgia and I was discharged from the hospital.

As far as I know no evidence was ever found that I had recently had a virus but I was pleased with this diagnosis, as it appeared to indicate that my strength should soon return and that there was no sinister cause.

Noticing that I was no better than when I was sent to hospital my G.P. started to visit once a week. I asked him if perhaps I had M.E. and his reply was "is there such a thing?" No other explanation or theory was offered.

During one of the G.P.'s early visits he prescribed pills (Triptafen). When I read the accompanying pamphlet I was horrified to find that these were anti-depressants. I certainly was not depressed and did not wish to be given that label.

When Colin returned home from work I was so upset that he arranged to see the G.P. to find out more about these pills. The G.P. explained that he thought that I appeared anxious and that the pills only had a small content of the anti-depressant drug and that they would also work as a muscle relaxant.

It would have saved some worry if this had been explained to me.

What the G.P. did not seem to realise was that I most certainly was anxious when he visited because I wondered what he was going to say. I was perfectly calm when there were no doctors around.

After several weekly visits I decided there was no point in continuing with them as the doctor did not have any idea what had happened to me.

Sometimes I could walk a few feet, and other times I couldn't walk at all. If anything I was weakening further and if Colin was working away from the house, before leaving for work, he was preparing not only my breakfast but also a tray with my lunch and a flask of hot drinks, which he left by the bed. I could just about reach the toilet next to the bedroom unaided. If he was at home he would carry me into the lounge or conservatory.

We racked our brains trying to think of another avenue we could explore to find the cause of my problem, because on reflection we were not convinced by the hospital diagnosis.

Having explored and eliminated all the neurological causes Colin had begun to wonder if I could be unknowingly poisoning myself in some way, so he asked my G.P. if I could see another consultant who might know about these things. To try to speed things up we paid to see a consultant physician at one of the local private hospitals.

On arrival Colin dropped me at the entrance to the hospital. To reach the reception area I had a choice of walking up some steps or the wheelchair ramp. I thought that the ramp would be easier but it was like climbing Mount Everest and left me exhausted.

When I was called to be weighed the nurse soon realised by the speed, snail-like, and the effort I was having to put into walking across the room, that there was something very wrong. However I was determined to walk into the consulting room under my own steam.

My determination was rewarded by the consultant's first words, delivered in a derogatory tone, which were "what a curious gait". I wished that I had not bothered.

The consultant proceeded to take notes of the course of my illness so far, then carried out a basic examination on the couch. On completion he announced rather dismissively that he did not know what was wrong with me.

By the time I arrived home I was very weak. Colin had to carry me into the bedroom and put me into bed.

It felt as if the skin on my face had dropped. Apparently it also looked that way, as if the muscles on my face didn't have the strength to hold the skin up. This was to happen frequently.

We were disillusioned at the attitude displayed and the fact that the consultant did not suggest any new avenues to explore.

Time was passing, but we hoped that things would improve soon. I had a follow up visit to the Outpatients neurology clinic at the Infirmary in November where I was seen by a junior doctor who I had not met before. He did not know my history but expressed surprise at the anti-depressants I had been prescribed. However he did not suggest any alternative. I was discharged from the care of the clinic.

Christmas came and we noticed that my energy levels were very, very gradually increasing. I could walk to the kitchen, a couple of times a day, to make a drink even though the kettle felt as if it weighed a ton. My muscles were still twitching and I was still experiencing a lot of spasmodic pain in them.

Over the next few months we were really pleased as the improvement continued. I was managing to do more and more. A little dusting for ten minutes, making the bed or preparing a snack. Only one of these activities a day nevertheless it was a huge step forward.

The time came when I could set myself targets. I had not discussed this with anyone but it seemed the logical thing to do provided I only attempted to do things as and when I felt able.

Firstly I aimed to walk to the bird bath situated half way down the back garden, a distance of twenty-five yards, and back. The hardest obstacle to this goal was the incline from the lawn to the patio which only rises six inches. I was very aware that I was walking in a peculiar fashion. My legs felt out of control and very stiff, and I could hardly lift my feet.

Gradually I was able to increase the distance I could walk and the amount of housework I could tackle. By March, that is after seven months, I thought the end of all my troubles was in sight. I had improved drastically and could manage to walk a couple of hundred yards on the flat without collapsing with exhaustion.

After being housebound during the short grey days and the long dark nights of winter I started to think of going away. It was like a dream to be able to contemplate such a thing.

We decided that I was up to going away, but where could we go to find some spring sunshine and warmth? Somewhere where the sun's rays would not be too powerful as I have always been allergic to strong sunlight which makes my skin blister.

The final decision was to drive to the south of France towing the caravan which we had bought eighteen months earlier. This seemed like going from the sublime to the ridiculous to contemplate such a journey, but I was game for anything. I so desperately wanted to be normal.

Colin packed the caravan and we became very excited at the prospect of such an adventure.

The first night was spent in an old orchard near Dover, and we were up at the crack of dawn to catch the ferry to Calais. It had been a very cold night with a hard frost, but we had been warm in our bed.

I did not think that the journey from home to Dover, a distance of two hundred and fifty miles, had affected me until I boarded the ferry. The climb from the car deck to the passenger areas involved several sets of stairs and proved a major obstacle to me. Colin had to haul me up.

On arrival in Calais we immediately headed south down the motorway. Stopping every two hours for a drink and a rest we made steady progress, passing Lyons before stopping for the night in a motorway service area. Late the following afternoon we arrived at a campsite a few miles from Saint Tropez.

It was a few days before Easter and there were not very many caravans on the site, so we had plenty of choice of pitch among the trees. Unfortunately the pitches which faced directly on to the beach were taken.

Long leisurely days were spent pottering along the beach to the new development of Port Grimaud, doing the shopping, which included plenty of baguettes, or walking in the other direction to look at the new golf course and holiday homes which surrounded it.

I can remember commenting at the time that I don't recall ever having eaten so much bread when we had been to France before. Looking back this may have been a sign of the troubles to come but neither of us thought anything of it at the time.

Occasionally we would venture further afield and drive to Monaco or up into the hills where we would discover the small mountain villages with their brightly coloured flowers and narrow streets.

Over the Easter period the campsite became horrendously crowded with other caravans and tents pitching within a few feet of us. This was not at all relaxing but, fortunately, nearly everyone disappeared immediately after the Easter break.

Walking round the site and down to the shore we were amazed to find several empty plots virtually on the beach, so we hurried back to our caravan and moved to one of those.

We stayed in this position, overlooking the Mediterranean, until it was time to set off on our homeward journey. Three lovely relaxing weeks had passed very quickly and things were looking good.

To break the journey home we stopped in Annecy, where we stayed several days.

I was surprised how much I had improved, so much so that on the odd occasion I walked a mile or so. I was better, or so I thought.

CHAPTER 2

Over the summer months life was more or less normal. I had gradually weaned myself off the anti-depressants, which was a relief, as I did not like the side effect of a very dry mouth.

I had also gained two stone in weight which I attributed to the pills, but noticed that this did not disappear. As I am only five feet tall and normally weigh eight stone the extra weight was particularly noticeable.

None of my clothes would fit so I had to buy some new ones, but not many as I was determined to lose the extra weight as soon as possible. This was to take a lot longer than expected, as it proved very difficult to get to the bottom of the reason for the gain.

August 1994 was lovely and sunny and as I had been feeling really strong for several months I decided to decorate the dining room.

Browsing through a women's magazine I noticed an advertisement for an interesting new concept in wallpapers, which Marks and Spencers was selling. The paper was self-adhesive, no pasting or soaking in water. I thought I would try it as I have always enjoyed decorating.

The nearest Marks and Spencers which sold the wallpaper was at the Meadowhall development, an hours drive away, so off I went. I very much liked the look and texture of the paper so ended up buying some for the bedroom as well as the dining room.

A few days later Colin and I started to paper the dining room. Colin assisted by cutting the paper to the required length and I hung it. We soon finished the job and I didn't feel too bad. No worse than I used to after wall papering even though it was about twenty-two degrees outside.

After a couple of days rest I decided I would like to tackle the bedroom. This we did but I noticed I was increasingly finding it a strain to climb the step ladders with each successive piece of wallpaper, and the heat was not helping matters. Nevertheless we were very pleased with the finished result, now I would rest for a few days.

It was not long before the dreadful truth dawned on us. Once again I was completely exhausted. Never mind, I was sure it would only be a matter of days before my strength returned.

I was soon to realise that I had been far too optimistic. It was to be weeks before I could manage on occasions to walk from room to room.

The extreme pain and twitching in my muscles returned and I toyed with the idea of going back on the antidepressants to try to calm my muscles.

I wasn't sure which was worse, the side effects of the pills or the pains.

I didn't know if the pills helped, but I decided to give them another go. I had read that they did not start to have any effect for two to three weeks so I would have to be patient.

By now it had become clear that a pattern was emerging of rest, gain a little strength, do too much, back to resting.

Being able to manage my small amount of energy was something I would find very difficult. Invariably I would do far too much when I felt good.

This happened for two reasons. Firstly the sheer pleasure of being able to achieve some small task after so long made me think I was stronger than I was. Secondly I couldn't tell the difference between tiredness and exhaustion until it was too late. Everyone found it hard to believe that I could keep overdoing things, but there were not any warning signs.

When I was exhausted I felt absolutely drained. It was as if my battery had gone flat. It was certainly not lack of motivation which rendered me incapable of functioning.

I now realize that I never yawned when I was exhausted. I was way past the point at which you would normally yawn.

I very rarely stayed in bed all day. Colin would usually carry me, if I could not manage to walk, to the conservatory where I would sit or lie watching the wildlife in the garden or sleeping.

We are very fortunate in that we have a lovely garden with lots of species of trees and shrubs which encourage many different types of wildlife. There are usually two female and one male pheasants, red legged partridges, too many rabbits because they eat the plants, squirrels and numerous types of birds.

On a good day I was able to watch the birds through the binoculars for several minutes, if I was strong enough to hold them up. I also enjoyed watching the leaves bursting into life in the spring, particularly on the silver birch tree.

The passing of time was not really noticeable day to day as the routine was exactly the same. Have a bath, lie down, eat the meals Colin cooked for me, go to bed. No physical or mental stimulation as neither my mind nor body was up to that.

We now thought I must have M.E. and read every article we could find on the subject and I joined the M.E. Association. Their magazines are full of interesting articles.

Friends and family also read or listened to any relevant programmes and passed on the information. One piece in the newspaper suggested that taking a drug called sertraline might help so I mentioned this to the doctor and tried it, but it was to no avail.

Not everyone was so supportive. Some acquaintances said ridiculous things which were very hurtful, and which I could well have done without.

One person suggested the cause of my troubles was the fact that we had been burgled. One day, before I was ill, I had come home from shopping and noticed, as I drove up to the front door, that there was a branch of a fuschia bush on the lawn. I wondered how that had got there.

As we had been burgled twice before I went next door and asked a friend if she would accompany me while I opened the door and went in. This she did and immediately we noticed a large window in the hall had been smashed. There was glass all over the floor and some blood but there wasn't anyone in the house. The jewelry I had left from the previous burglaries had been taken this time, including family inheritances. I was not particularly disturbed by this as there was nothing I could do about it.

Very occasionally I would have a reasonably good day and Colin would suggest going for a ride out in the car for a change of scene. Not too far, perhaps to the local nursery to look at the plants and have a cup of coffee.

It was on one of these occasions that we met someone who we had known for a long time. We had a brief chat and she suggested I might feel better if I got myself a job. This really upset me as that remark left me in no doubt what she thought was the cause of my problem.

Colin told me to forget it as these people were not worth getting upset over, but to this day I get upset when I think about it.

My son and daughter-in-law have three boys, who at this time were aged one, three and five, and live in Birmingham. Consequently we could not see them unless they came to visit us because it was a two hour journey to their house and was too far for me to travel.

The grandchildren are normal, healthy, boisterous children so we had to limit their visits to one child at a time and, depending on how I was, put a time limit on their stay. This unfortunately was usually only about ten minutes before I felt absolutely exhausted. I knew we were missing them growing up and all the developments children make at that age.

As with most families today all our relations are spread around the country but we were in constant touch over the telephone. I would talk if I was able, if not Colin would keep them informed of progress or lack of it.

Friends were very supportive and eager to help but as Colin was at home there was not much they could do. At first I would try to speak to everyone who 'phoned but we soon had to make the decision to limit my chats as it was far too tiring. Most of the time I could manage ten minutes once every five days or so. They all recognised that there was something very wrong because they knew my fondness for chatting, and that I would not be staying in the house if I could possibly be out and about.

I was making arrangements for friends to come to see me but Colin always had to cancel the visit. Eventually I realized that I could not live as before and would have to live one day at a time and not consider the future. I had no idea what the future held.

The support our friends gave to Colin was equally important. I was keen that he should go to play golf with his golfing pals on a Saturday morning. If I was too ill to be left on my own my daughter would sit with me. I felt it was important for him to have a change of scene and to get away from the stressful situation.

We very rarely had an unbroken night's sleep. I was in a lot of pain and painkillers did not help at all, so my tossing and turning would wake him up numerous times a night. We drank endless cups of tea and spent a lot of time going round in circles, wondering where to turn for help.

At one time Colin bought a book on back problems because at first glance it looked as if it had some relevant information.

Having digested its contents we decided that it contained the answer. My problem was due to pressure on certain points of my neck. These points should be massaged to relieve the pressure, so Colin rushed out to buy a massager. He massaged my spine, neck and shoulders every morning. This identified swollen painful areas and was very soothing but after a few weeks there was no noticeable improvement.

It was to be a long time before I found out what was causing the swelling.

I had heard and read about reflexology and knew of a lady who was a qualified reflexologist so this was to be the next avenue I would explore. I found it fascinating and had treatment for several months but did not feel that this made any improvement in my condition.

We were rapidly running out of ideas. Acupuncture, hypnotism, herbal and Chinese medicine and any other form of alternative therapy were not appealing to me, although I suspected that in the end I may come to try them as by now I was absolutely determined to find the cause of my illness, and a cure.

CHAPTER 3

In September 1995, two years after the onset of my ill health, I became weaker than at any previous time. Complete bed rest became my way of life apart from being helped to the bathroom, which is off the bedroom.

I enjoyed a daily bath, as lying in the warm water seemed to help the pains in my muscles as well as making me feel refreshed. Colin would run the water, help with my ablutions and dry me, then assist with putting on my pyjamas.

I would collapse on the bed from the exertion and have to have my legs lifted up and put into the resting position. Having been tucked up I would lie completely motionless, unable to speak, lift a finger, or even move my eyes.

It would be at least a couple of hours before I would be able to manage, with Colin's assistance, to have a drink or to eat a few mouthfuls of food. After doing so I would need to lie motionless again.

Slowly over the following weeks I regained some strength and Colin would carry me into the lounge, if I could not walk there, where I would lie on the settee.

By this time Colin was becoming an expert at housekeeping and being a carer but now confesses that, naturally, he was very worried about my state of health. He decided to pay the G.P. a visit to request a second opinion from another neurologist. He also asked that this should be a home consultation. The only reason we asked for a neurologist was because we still could not think of any other branch of medicine to explore and the G.P. had not suggested any different speciality.

When the neurologist arrived he asked for a history of my illness, then asked me to lie on the bed while he did some tests on the strength of my muscles.

Some of these tests involved pushing as hard as I could against his hands with the soles of my feet. I could do this quite well. What he did not realize was that, at this stage, I could manage to respond to these light tests. The dreadful weakness was when my body had to move its own weight.

Basically the neurologist said that I had had all the electrical tests and the results had been O.K. He would try a new test as a last resort although he did not expect to find anything wrong. I would then have to look to the cause of my problem being psychological.

When he had gone we just looked at each other and said what a waste of time and money that had been. We were both upset at his attitude but it was not entirely unexpected. I would have the test just in case it came up with anything. By now I was becoming anti-doctor.

I was apprehensive when I went for the test. I explained my symptoms to yet another doctor and also that I had started to have what felt like electric shocks on my arms. I was soon put in my place and told that I wasn't a doctor and didn't know that they were shocks. I kept quiet but for years I have had shocks when touching the car, and these sensations were like much stronger versions of those.

To prepare for the test I had to sit with my feet in a bowl of hot water until my feet were very warm. My hands were already warm. Then I had to lie on the couch and have needles inserted into my muscles. An electric current was then passed through the needles into the muscles and the results came up on a computer screen. The strength of current was far greater than any I had experienced before and was very painful.

While the test was being done the doctor asked me some more questions and I explained that I had been ill for a long time. His reply was "I bet your G.P. was sick of seeing you".

I was absolutely amazed and lost for words. Before I left he told me that the test was negative.

I couldn't get out of there fast enough and when I saw Colin I immediately burst into tears and begged him not to make me see any more doctors. I felt totally humiliated and this was the last straw.

Colin had a tough time trying to buoy up my spirits. Fortunately he is always on an even keel and he told me again that these people were not worth wasting precious energy over.

Several friends received tearful 'phone calls at this time and they were all astonished at what this particular doctor had said. I found talking and crying over these incidences helped me get them out of my system, otherwise I would have dwelt on them for a long time.

The more I thought about the incident, the more I felt compelled to act. I wondered who exactly doctors think they are that they can speak to people in this way. Particularly as you are only seeing them as there is something wrong, and you are not at your strongest, otherwise you would not be there.

I was so furious that I decided to send a letter of complaint to the hospital via the Community Health Council, of which I was a member until I became ill. The complaints officer came to see me and to hear my story, and together we drafted a letter to set the procedure in motion. (The government has since scrapped Community Health Councils.)

In reality I knew that nothing would be done, and I was correct, but at least the letter of complaint will be on file. The official response from the hospital stated that the doctor did not realize he had upset me. Not exactly a satisfactory outcome but at least I felt a little better in retaliating.

The next we heard was a telephone call for Colin from our G.P. asking him to go and see him. We could guess what this would be about. He must have had a letter from the neurologist. We were sure he was going to say that the test results were negative, and that the neurologist had suggested I should see a psychiatrist as the cause of my illness could be psychological.

When Colin came home he had a grin on his face and we both had a good laugh. We had been correct. Colin's reply to this suggestion was that we did not accept the diagnosis and that I would not be seeing any psychiatrists. Back to square one.

Another few months passed without

me seeing any doctors because I had been completely put off doing so. It appeared to me that members of the medical profession did not believe what I said. With their attitude they had totally destroyed my self-confidence. I felt very low mentally and utterly miserable. In my view it was akin to being sent to prison when innocent.

I was having great difficulty sleeping and sometimes my heart not beating rhythmically would wake me. It wasn't racing or thudding or missing a beat, it was almost as if it was fluttering. It is very hard to describe exactly how it felt but it made me feel very light headed.

I had shocks all over my body, but worst of all were the ones all over my scalp, very severe pains and twitches in all muscles, not just arms and legs, from which there was no relief. The muscle at the top of my left arm felt as if it had a clamp round it and the pain was excruciating. I had been given Diazepam but did not find it eased the agony at all. I did not know where to put my arm.

Sometimes the twitches in my leg muscles were so strong that they made my whole body shake. The small muscles around my nose and mouth twitched constantly. I felt like a rabbit.

I was cold all the time but it was particularly noticeable in bed. A few minutes after lying down I would suddenly become extremely cold right through to the core. I felt as if I was shivering deep inside and I took ages to thaw out. Fleecy pyjamas and a hot water bottle became necessary even in the summer. During the day my hands and feet were never warm.

After some thought we wondered if this might be a sign of low blood pressure. Every time I had my blood pressure taken it had been normal so we discounted that.

One night I had a terrible pain in my side which I had not experienced before and I was slightly worried about this so we called the doctor. As it was out of surgery hours a doctor we did not know came. She was very sympathetic and said that it was a muscle vacillating, that is twitching.

Painkillers were suggested but I knew from experience that if it was a muscle twitching violently painkillers would not offer any relief. The twitching occurred several times that night and was so strong that it made the bed shake. I found this traumatic and we really wondered what on earth was happening to me.

Sometimes when very weak I would have to lie down after eating, because my heart would be thudding and I would feel light headed. This was a completely different sensation to the one I sometimes had in the night when my heart wasn't beating regularly.

After about an hour I would feel a bit better. I could only assume this was because my body was using what small amount of energy I had to digest the food but I now know differently.

My throat had been feeling very strange for a long time. It was not sore but I was having great difficulty swallowing. I did not like this sensation at all. Sometimes it was slightly easier to swallow than other times but it was never normal. I noticed that it seemed to be worse after drinking. Eventually I came to the conclusion that there must be something in the water to which I was reacting.

Colin bought a water filter of the jug variety which made a big difference to start with. My throat didn't feel as though it was swollen after using the filtered water, for both drinking and cooking for a couple of months, but then it became just as bad as it had been before.

I telephoned an allergy clinic to find out what sort of water filter they used and purchased the same type. This had to be installed under the sink, which Colin did, and a tap fitted on to the draining board. Since I have been drinking this water only I have not had a swollen throat. On holiday I buy bottled water but have found some types of those affect me.

I had a sore tongue with edges that looked as if a mouse had taken chunks out of it, cracks, smooth patches and sometimes it would bleed. It was very painful when eating. I also had dry eyes and tiny red spots had started appearing all over my body. My skin had lost its colour. My G.P. noticed this and compared the palm of my hand with his. Mine was white and his was pink.

A rash had appeared on my neck a long time before I was ever ill. It just looked like a big red blotch which covered the whole of the front of my neck. It didn't itch and it was there continuously. Later on I developed rashes on my arms, sometimes these itched and they tended to become worse when I was in the bath or when hot. Occasionally my torso would be completely covered in a rash.

Lying in bed it was very noticeable that I had a high pitched noise in my ear which was there all the time. It didn't matter which side I lay on or if I was sitting up, it was still there. There wasn't any pain just an irritating continuous noise. I would have this for weeks on end and then it would disappear only to return again. I assumed that this was tinnitus but never mentioned it to any member of the medical profession.

I had become very sensitive to noise. This sensitivity was most intense when I was at my weakest. The slightest noise frightened me. Even though the floor is carpeted the very soft sound of Colin walking past the closed bedroom door was like a very loud noise to me. This made life even more difficult for him when he was trying to get some jobs done. I needed complete rest and quiet or I would end up feeling petrified, perspiring profusely, heart racing and tears streaming down my face. The stress of any sound was unbearable.

Lack of sleep was taking its toll. I was still taking the anti-depressants as I was sure they helped me get to sleep but I still woke frequently during the night.

When I became a little stronger the level of noise I could bear increased. During the day if I was up to it I would sometimes watch T.V. with the sound low, always programmes which didn't need any concentration and had pretty scenery. If I progressed to reading the newspaper things were really looking up.

I was asked many times if I got bored. Definitely not. Most of the time my brain simply would not function. I could not think straight or concentrate. I felt very fuzzy headed. It was amazing how quickly the time passed at every stage of incapacity.

My appetite varied according to my strength, sometimes I would have to be coaxed to eat a small amount, but Colin was gently insistent. He would always prepare very varied and nutritious meals, and it was fortuitous that he did. This has proved to be crucial.

CHAPTER 4

After being housebound for months I remember well the first time Colin took me out in the car to the local market town. It is a journey of ten miles through the local countryside.

To see the trees and fields was so exciting. I was like a child at Christmas. The colours were so vivid and it was as if everything was jumping out at me. The traffic seemed to be moving so quickly, it was quite frightening.

Another simple day to day occurrence left me totally unsure of myself, that of handling money. It took some time to get used to working out simple addition of prices and the value of the coins and notes. This was particularly difficult if I was in a queue and felt under pressure to hurry. I would end up asking Colin to pay.

Three years had passed now but I started to notice that once again I was very gradually regaining some strength until I reached the point where I decided that I would be able to make the journey to the Lake District. We took the caravan and stayed on a site near Coniston.

A few days were spent just sitting by the lake or walking a few yards for a bit of gentle exercise. Inevitably one day I thought that I could do more than I could.

The distance to the caravan from where we had been sitting was about half a mile and I was sure that I would be able to manage to make it back to the site. By taking my time and walking very slowly I arrived back unaided, albeit exceedingly tired. Unfortunately the next morning the awful truth dawned on us. I hardly had the energy to sit up.

It was back to square one once again. We had to go home and go back to the old routine of spending most of the day lying down having my meals brought to me and generally being looked after.

While we were away I had noticed a change in bowel habits. I was passing bulky stools. This I ignored for a few months because I put it down to being just another symptom.

Eventually I went to the surgery but saw another doctor, not my usual G.P., who suggested that I went for an abdominal scan. This did not show anything untoward but I was told that I had a fatty liver. I did not know what this meant, there was no explanation given but I was asked if I drank a lot of alcohol. I have never been keen on alcohol, only drinking the very occasional glass of wine.

A couple of weeks later I went to see my own G.P. who said that he would not have sent me for the scan but that he would refer me to a gastroenterologist.

After a few weeks I received an appointment with the gastro-enterologist. He ordered a blood test and a biopsy of the intestines but gave no reason for either of these tests nor explained what he was testing for. The atmosphere in the clinic was so rushed that patients were not encouraged to ask questions.

I went for the biopsy. This involved swallowing a tube, with tiny snippers on the end, so that a small piece of intestine could be taken for examination. A sedative can be given for this, if requested, so that there is no difficulty swallowing the tube.

The doctor who was administering the sedative said that they were looking for coeliac disease. This is an allergy to gluten which is the protein in wheat which gives dough its elasticity. Gluten is also in oats, barley and rye.

A biopsy is the definitive test for coeliac disease although there is now a blood test which a G.P. can do as a preliminary test.

The inside of the intestines consist of tiny protrusions, called villi, through which nutrients from foods are absorbed. If a coeliac eats gluten the effect on the villi is such that they flatten resulting in malabsorption. In babies this is known as failure to thrive. Surely this is what I was doing.

Many people do not experience bowel symptoms such as I did but have one or more chronic ailments. Among some of the more common syptoms are anaemia, tiredness, diarrhoea, stomach bloating and pain, loss of weight and osteoporosis.

Coeliac Disease is becoming more common. In Ireland the incidence is between 1 in 100 and 1 in 150 of the population. Recent studies have indicated that the rate in the U.K. is probably far greater than the 1 in 1000 to 1 in 300 than had been previously thought.

The wheat that is imported today has a higher gluten content than other wheat and it is thought that this is the reason for the increase in the incidence.

When I saw the gastroenterologist again he explained that the biopsy confirmed that I was coeliac. The advice given was that I must stay off gluten for the rest of my life and for further information I should make an appointment with the hospital dietician.

A further biopsy would be carried out when I had been on the gluten free diet for three months to see if the villi had recovered.

I saw the hospital dietician a couple of weeks later but did not receive much useful help. Basically I was told to join the Coeliac Society, this has now been renamed Coeliac UK, which I did, and I was given some leaflets.

The society publish regular magazines containing interesting articles and recipes, and a book which is updated each year with lists of foods which are gluten free, and their manufacturers. There is also a list of all the items such as bread, flour and biscuits which can be obtained on prescription. I also joined the local branch of the society.

Once again we avidly read anything from any source to find out as much information on the subject as we could. I was very pleased with the diagnosis, surely if I made sure that I never ate gluten again I would soon be better.

I was horrified when I realized that I was not back to my old self after several months on the gluten free diet. The follow up biopsy had shown that my villi had recovered. It was obvious that the diagnosis of Coeliac Disease was not going to be the final answer to my problems. No such luck.

Sticking to the coeliac diet is not as easy as it sounds as gluten is in many foods which I would never have thought of, and eating out is a minefield. Probably the hardest thing is trying to find a snack to eat in a cafe when out and about, as most snacks in this country tend to be wheat based.

Cross contamination is also a risk. In a cafe it is very easy to eat food prepared on a surface that has already had gluten containing foods touching it.

Reading labels when shopping, and sticking to plain cooking in a restaurant is a must.

About this time there was a new development. I started to wake in the night feeling very agitated, sweating profusely and needing to eat, in particular I needed carbohydrate. I had no idea why this was. I would potter around at least once and sometimes twice a night wondering what on earth I could eat now that I was on this restricted gluten-free diet. More often than not I would end up eating some rice with fruit.

After this had been going on for some weeks I was beginning to feel very tired, very low mentally and as if I could not cope. My sister has suffered with hypoglycaemia, low blood sugar, for years and I suspected that I now had the same problem.

CHAPTER 5

While waiting to see the gastroenterologist for the results of the biopsy to ascertain whether I was coeliac, I decided that I would have a hysterectomy.

I had known for years before I was ill that I had a large fibroid but as it wasn't giving me any trouble I was perfectly happy not to have surgery. The doctors I had seen about my mysterious symptoms had all expressed surprise, when they had been examining my stomach, at the size of the lump and suggested I would be better off without it.

I wasn't at all worried about having the operation as I was relatively strong at this time and hoped I may show signs of improvement after the fibroid had been removed.

The operation went very well and a fibroid the size of a melon was

Blood test for allergies

removed along with my ovaries and fallopian tubes. So that I would not suffer hormonal complications I had a hormone implant.

I was sent out of hospital on the fifth day and recovered as quickly as anybody would after a hysterectomy. The operation did not effect my other problems at all, or vice versa.

While I was in hospital my daughter brought me some magazines one of which contained an article on food allergies. It explained that a simple blood test could detect allergies, although it required sending a sample to the United States.

The symptoms described in the article fitted a lot of my own symptoms so I decided that I would have this test. It was pretty expensive at £200 but I thought that it was an avenue worth exploring.

When I received the results I was amazed to see that I was allergic to several foods. These allergies are not life threatening and are sometimes referred to as sensitivities by some members of the medical profession.

The foods highlighted in the test as showing a reaction were banana, green beans, melon, cheese, pepper, egg, milk, mushroom, pea, potato, rye, safflower, wheat, and baker's and brewer's yeast.

I was not at all surprised to see milk and cheese on the list of allergies as I had already noticed that when I ate these my throat, neck and face swelled.

One night I couldn't get to sleep. I felt exceedingly agitated and had been tossing and turning for ages so in the end I thought I would go and read in the lounge. It didn't take long to realize that I couldn't sit still never mind read or watch the television. All I could do was pace up and down, I must have been running on adrenaline, I just did not know what to do with myself.

Rotation diet – 5 day

The agitated feeling lasted all night and during the morning. Eventually as the day wore on I started to calm down and we tried to work out what had been the cause of my feeling that way.

The only possible reason we could come up with was that it might have been the effect of having eaten some cheese with the evening meal. I never ate cheese or drank milk again and didn't have the same reaction until much later when other foods began to have a similar effect.

Some literature was sent with the test results explaining about rotation diets and food families. This was an entirely new area about which I knew nothing. It all seemed very strange and there was a lot to learn.

The aim of a rotation diet is that no food or food family should be eaten more often than every five days so that the allergic reaction is lessened.

Eventually Colin sat down, sorted all the foods I was eating into their food families, worked out some diet sheets following the guidelines in the literature and printed them off the computer.

The diet sheets were stuck on to the front of the kitchen cupboard doors where I could refer to them every time I had a meal.

As many foods and as much as required may be eaten from the allowed foods for that day.

Below is an example of my diet for meat and fish: -

Day 1	Day 2	Day 3	Day 4
Turkey	Lamb	Beef	Rabbit
Chicken	Cod	Venison	Plaice
Duck	Haddock	Sardines	Ostrich
Pheasant	Pork	Salmon	Prawns

Rotation diet = New lease of energy

By having everything I was eating sorted into families and by sticking to this rigidly, I noticed a new found lease of energy.

It was a nuisance always having to think about food and entailed an awful lot more shopping. Normally if some meat was left over from one day to the next it would be eaten but now we had to try to buy just the required amount for one meal, otherwise Colin would end up eating leftovers all the time. Nevertheless the hassle was worth it as I was noticeably stronger.

Another sign which convinced me that foods were playing a large part in my problems was that I lost some weight very quickly after starting to follow the rotation diet, but nowhere near all of the two stone I had gained. This was even though I was eating normal size portions of carbohydrate, protein and fats as this was not a diet in the sense of a weight loss diet.

The large lumps above my collar bone were still noticeable, my whole body was pretty swollen and the back of my shoulders were very painful. It was several years before I found out that the pain and swelling was caused by fluid.

CHAPTER 6

I had a hospital appointment, at the coeliac clinic, at a time when I was really struggling to walk. For some unknown reason I had relapsed. This time I saw a lady doctor, whom I had not seen before, who expressed concern that I was on the point of collapse after having only walked a few yards.

She gave me a thorough examination, the most thorough I have ever had. She was very sympathetic and wanted to admit me to hospital immediately for further tests to try to get to the bottom of some of my troubles, but there was not a free bed.

I told her that I had lots of allergies and showed her the list of them but she did not pass any comment.

A week later I was admitted to hospital for tests. By now I was thoroughly fed up with hospitals, doctors and nurses but steeled myself for what was to come.

I was in hospital for several days during which time I had a CT scan of my abdomen and among other things a barium endoscopy. For this test a tube has to be swallowed which is then passed through the stomach into the intestine, the barium liquid is poured down the tube and its progress is observed on a screen.

I was so weak when having these tests that they were no problem as I could not have cared less about anything that was happening to me. I could not resist at all. I didn't even have the strength to hold my head up. The nurses suggested that I was too weak to have the tests but I just wanted to get them over.

When I was having the endoscopy the doctor said that they had found something on my small intestine but

Stomach upset after gluten contaminated chicken

that he had no idea what it was. Fortunately it was nothing more serious than an adhesion from the hysterectomy, but it required stomach surgery a few weeks later to ascertain this.

Once again I explained about the allergies and rashes and other symptoms I had, although I did not go into full details as clearly the doctors did not want to know. They gave the impression that they were losing their patience with me.

Most of the time Colin prepared and brought my food from home however I risked eating a hospital meal of chicken. This was a big mistake as I suffered a severe stomach upset. I suspected the chicken was the culprit so Colin went to the hospital kitchen to see how the chicken had been cooked. All the food was bought in frozen and heated. The method of heating the chicken was to deep fat fry it. Other food which had been coated in breadcrumbs had been fried in the same fat thereby causing contamination with gluten. After I stopped eating the chicken my stomach recovered.

I had a lot of blood tests at this time and I asked the consultant what the tests were for. I was told that there were far too many to explain.

I also had a muscle biopsy to see if they could find anything wrong with my muscles. I am so glad I did not know in advance what having a muscle biopsy entailed. Needles of varying lengths were inserted to different depths into a thigh muscle to take samples for testing. Out of all the tests I had endured this was by far the most painful. I think a sedative should have been given.

A few weeks later I saw the consultant again and he advised that all the tests were clear. When I said that "the tests may be okay but I was not okay" he told me to "go and get on with living. You have a leaky gut, are coeliac and have M.E.".

It was stated that if there were any nutritional deficiencies they would be made up in five weeks. This has been proved to be completely wrong in my case.

I definitely did not think that I had a specific illness called M.E. Yes I had what are recognised as M.E. symptoms but my personal opinion is that M.E. is an umbrella term for unexplained debilitating illness whatever the cause. The cause or causes may vary from person to person.

Leaky gut. What on earth is that? I had never heard of it, but the consultant said that would be the cause of my allergies. No remedy was offered.

As for getting on with living, he clearly did not understand that I did not want to be and would not be sitting around, or often lying around all day if I could be doing something.

Since then I have read that a leaky gut is when there are tiny holes in the intestines which allow minute particles of partly digested food into the blood system thereby causing allergies to develop. In my case undiagnosed coeliac disease was more than likely the cause of my leaky gut and therefore also the cause of my allergies.

It was obvious that I was going to have to obtain more information about food allergies but it was very difficult to know where to turn for advice.

Then one day I heard of a laboratory not far away that specialised in blood tests similar to the one I had sent to America. I thought it would be interesting to have the tests to see how the results compared with the American results. The only foods which appeared on both lists as positive were yeast, milk and egg.

> 3 years food diary
> challenge and reaction

Another way of trying to determine which foods were affecting me was to keep a food diary. For three years I wrote down everything, food or liquid, that passed my lips and the reactions I experienced. When I had been doing this for two years no clear pattern had emerged, so I began to wonder if it could be possible that everything I was eating was making me ill.

Around this time I saw another dietician, this time privately, in the hope that I might obtain some help with my allergies. Basically she did not believe a lot of what I said, particularly anything to do with my allergy tests, as she said that everyone who had them more or less had the same results.

She told me to drink some milk and to eat the foods I had a problem with, according to the tests, to see what happened. I was very reluctant do so and was not at all surprised when my face and neck swelled and other

cravings and offending foods

symptoms such as muscle pains and twitches returned. There was no point in continuing this relationship.

I also saw a dietician at the surgery and she was sceptical about the number of foods I thought were affecting me. Once again I came to the conclusion that it would be better to try to sort myself out.

It is amazing how long it takes to work out anything related to food. Apart from feeling shaky and sweating when my blood sugar was low, I also had the same symptoms with cravings. It is not a wonder I felt terrible when I had both causing the shakiness and sweating at the same time. In effect a double dose.

Corn, rice, chocolate, nuts and sugar produced the worst cravings. I would notice that I was feeling slightly agitated and this would intensify until I would feel really bad tempered, start sweating and shaking. Off I would trot

sweating, shaking, palpitations, agitated, insomnia

to the kitchen to eat the offending food. I always knew which food I was craving as my brain didn't seem to be able to think about anything else. Within a couple of minutes of eating I would be sweating more profusely and my heart would be thudding. Eventually this wore off and calm came over me.

Not being able to sleep was driving us potty. I would toss and turn all night. If I wasn't strong enough to get out of bed to get a drink, which was frequently, Colin would be having to get up several times a night to fetch one for me. This would sometimes go on for weeks.

I would be upset and we would lie in bed talking things over, going round and round in circles. What was happening to me? Where could we turn for help? Why couldn't I sleep?

Eventually I would give in and start taking 10mg. of Triptafen again. It was a case of which was worse, not being able to sleep or having to drink all the time because of the side effects of a dry mouth.

Every time I went through a weak phase I would take the pills for several months to help with the sleep problem. They helped me to go to sleep but I would still wake several times in the night. I didn't take them when stronger as I slept reasonably well.

For the first time I had lost a lot of weight and my bones were protruding. This combined with the amount of time spent lying down meant that it was becoming increasingly difficult to find a painless resting position. My hips, ankles, buttocks and heels were the most painful.

We thought about buying a new mattress but there really wasn't anything wrong with the present one. The answer we came up with in the end was to put a thick single duvet on top *private allergy and nutritional doctor*

of the mattress on my side of the bed and to lie on that. It wasn't perfect but it offered some relief.

My friends were still telephoning although I only had the strength to talk occasionally for a few minutes. One day a friend rang to say that she had heard of a young girl with similar problems to myself who had been seeing a private doctor, who specialised in nutritional and allergy treatments, and whose practice was only twenty miles away from home.

It did not take me long to decide that I would like to go and see this doctor.

So that I was able to undertake the journey we fully reclined the front seat in the car and put a pillow on the headrest. Even so the movement of the car and being jiggled around made me feel unbearably ill. It took forty five minutes to arrive at the clinic by which time I could not move, so we would park in the nearby supermarket car park until I regained a little strength and could be helped into reception.

The one hour consultation consisted of the history of my health throughout my life but especially since I became ill in 1993. The physical examination was to look at my nails, the skin on my hands, my tongue and the inside of my mouth. The state of these can show whether there are any nutritional deficiencies.

On the basis of my medical history and the examination it was suggested I should take some multi-vitamin and mineral supplements.

Immediately after the consultation I had an intravenous drip feed of a cocktail of nutrients to try to boost my energy levels quickly. I came out of the clinic feeling exhausted but with high hopes because at last I had found a doctor who believed every word I said and offered some hope of a recovery.

I cannot say that I noticed any improvement in my energy levels after the first drip. It had been suggested that regular intravenous drips of vitamins and minerals would be a good idea so I travelled to have these every two weeks, for several visits, as well as taking the supplements. Each visit was a mammoth excursion and unsurprisingly it took days to recover.

After a few months on the new regime plus the rotation diet I started to feel considerably stronger and able to do things which I had not been able to do for a long time.

Desensitising injections for my allergies had been advised but I really did not feel up to starting the treatment at that time, as I was not sure if these injections might possibly make me feel worse. I left the decision in abeyance for the time being.

At one point I was so well that I hardly had to lie down during the day at all. This prompted us to discuss going abroad in January for some sunshine.

We booked a holiday in an apartment in Majorca so that we could do our own catering as it would be much easier to cope with the difficulties of the gluten free diet and of the rotation diet, which I was still following for the allergies.

The walking at the airport was going to be a problem so we booked a wheelchair. I found the journey exceptionally tiring so as soon as we reached the apartment I went straight to bed.

A couple of days resting in the apartment was needed to get over the journey but then we managed to go out for a little drive in the car for a couple of miles, or sit outside a pavement cafe, interspersed with afternoon sleeps. It was a lovely change of scene which brightened us both up.

CHAPTER 7

Life was considerably easier than it had been for a long time. I had now been taking the supplements for a year and there were very noticeable changes in my health.

Sometimes the nutritional treatment would have more supplements added according to my symptoms. I always took Vitamin C, multi-vitamins and minerals, and a combination of evening primrose oil and fish oil. Later on selenium, copper and zinc, eventually calcium, magnesium, potassium and chromium were also added.

All the supplements were free of all common allergens and very high dose, stronger than the recommended daily allowance for a healthy adult. Sometimes I worried slightly about the fact that I was taking so many pills at such high doses, but if severely deficient this is what is required and I was under medical supervision.

Chronic fatigue can be a result of nutritional deficiencies caused by other factors such as stress, poor diet, allergies, illness or medical conditions related to the intestines or bowel which cause malabsorption.

I think my deficiencies were a result of having been coeliac for a long time before diagnosis thereby causing malnutrition. Unfortunately late diagnosis is common and is something I cannot comprehend when a simple blood test is all it would take to rule out coeliac disease.

Colin is a good example of how stress can leave you nutritionally deficient. He started to feel exceedingly tired, particularly when cutting the grass, playing golf and walking anywhere. I noticed he had to keep sitting on the garden seat for rests when gardening and told him that this was not normal at his age, at the time he was fifty-two years old.

I tried to persuade him to see the nutritional doctor but he kept insisting that he was perfectly alright. When he started to struggle to get round the golf course he decided he would seek help.

After several months on high strength multi-vitamin and mineral supplements, zinc, selenium and evening primrose and fish oil capsules there was a huge improvement in his energy levels.

Obviously the strain of the past few years had taken their toll on his health, which was not at all surprising. He now tells me that when I spent long periods lying down in an exceptionally weak state he thought that I was dying.

The fact that there wasn't anyone he could talk to constructively about my health created an enormous strain on him.

Zinc

My hair, eyebrows and eyelashes had been falling out since I had been ill. The brush was always full of hairs, there were hairs on the pillow and bedding, my clothes and the furniture. My hair had receded about one inch on either side of the temples like a man's and had become very dry and wiry.

I had hoped that the hair loss would stop when I had been taking the supplements for some time and was disappointed when it hadn't.

I had been taking zinc with all the other pills after meals then one day I read in a book that it should be taken on an empty stomach to be most effective, so I started to take the zinc last thing at night.

Knowing that results from treating severe nutritional deficiencies with vitamins and minerals are not instantaneous I was pleased to notice that after a couple of months of taking

Candida
Zinc

zinc at night my eyelashes had stopped falling out.

Some time later the hairs on the bedding and clothes became much less until eventually there were no more. After several months there was some slight re-growth on my temples. My hair loss had upset me so to see the new soft downy hairs was very exciting. I assumed that the re-growth would continue until my hair was back to its former thickness. This was not to be the case.

My stomach had been reacting in a peculiar way for many months. Every time I ate anything it sounded as if it was fizzing. This was not the same as wind and turned out to be candida which is an overgrowth of yeast in the guts. To clear this I took a course of Diflucan.

I no longer had to get up in the night to eat to alleviate the hypoglycaemic symptoms and I had been sleeping easily without Triptafen for months.

My tongue wasn't cracked with smooth patches, my senses of taste and smell had returned, my limbs and muscles still hurt but not to the same extent as before, my lips were not peeling as much, the candida had cleared.

I could occasionally potter down the road for the paper, a distance of 200 yards. If I attempted this Colin would accompany me as sometimes I would completely grind to a halt, unable to walk another step and he would have to fetch the car to take me home.

If I was able to travel to the local town Colin would pull up outside the shop I wished to visit, and go and park the car. It was so exciting to be able to browse and catch up with the latest designs and colours in clothes. I would not buy anything but felt as if I had bought masses of new clothes such was the good feeling of being out and about.

On one occasion we went to the local shopping centre where it was possible to borrow a wheelchair. My clothes were all hanging off me at this time because of fluid loss so Colin suggested a trip to buy a few new items.

We went straight to a shop where we knew they sold casual clothes in bright colours. It was a mammoth task trying on tops and trousers but Colin and an assistant kept bringing items to the changing room.

It wasn't long before I completely ran out of energy and had to settle for some of the items I had managed to try on. Back into the wheelchair and home for several days rest, but gosh I felt good, and I was able to wear my new clothes while resting in the lounge.

Five years had passed and I still could not judge when I should have stopped doing something. I definitely needed to pace myself better for my own sanity as I felt very low mentally when I had to go back to lying down.

I had forgotten how bad the pain and weakness had been.

I was very frustrated even though there was a huge improvement in the time it took to regain a little strength. It would be days instead of months.

Several months later there was a new development which gave me a lot of pleasure. I noticed I had started to yawn. I was so excited because this was something I had not done for years. It started to tell me that I was getting very tired and it was time to stop whatever I was doing.

This was a huge leap forward. Now I knew when I had done enough and hopefully would not go past tiredness into exhaustion. It was still a fine line and inevitably I would topple over it occasionally.

I now decided I could face the

EPD

prospect of starting treatment for the allergies, but not for the allergy to gluten as this is a life long condition for which there is no cure.

The method of desensitising which the nutritional doctor uses is Enzyme Potentiated Desensitisation. A tiny dose of allergens, mixed with a natural enzyme which enhances the desensitisation, is injected just under the surface of the skin and repeated every two or three months to start with. The gap is increased as the symptoms improve. At the time of treatment known allergens must not be eaten or the treatment would not work.

When I had the first couple of injections I cut out the foods which I knew affected me, according to the results of the blood allergy test I had previously, but noticed that I felt much worse. I was warned that the injections could bring back all the old symptoms so assumed that this was why I felt so bad.

In fact, as was proved later, it turned out that I was actually allergic to far more foods than I could ever have imagined. I had not cut out enough foods, consequently the treatment was not working.

From thereon for future treatments I only ate kangaroo and yam for thirty-six hours around the time of the injection as I knew these foods would be safe. Dry fried kangaroo and boiled yam every mealtime including breakfast is no joke and I soon started to feel as if I couldn t swallow another mouthful.

Missing a meal was not an option because if I did I became like a rag doll and in a state of collapse.

For the next five days after the injection very tiny amounts, only a small spoonful, of many foods at each meal were allowed. After this period the amount of each food eaten could be increased until the amount which could

EPD side effects.
(withdrawal symptoms)?

be tolerated became obvious.

It was not easy to locate kangaroo and yam and Colin spent many hours driving round trying to find a supplier eventually finding a specialist meat wholesaler in the Midlands. By telephoning I managed to find a fruit and vegetable wholesaler who was willing to buy some yam from Covent Garden, but I would have to buy a box full. It took us ages to peel them as they are so slimy but eventually we blanched and froze them.

<u>Several times the treatment had disturbing side effects which took me totally by surprise.</u> I felt as if I couldn't carry on with the constant battles of all my problems any more. Suicidal thoughts kept coming into my head. I found no matter how hard I tried these thoughts would not go away.

At the time I thought that this was related to <u>withdrawal symptoms</u> from <u>corn and rice</u> because I had cut them

GPD side effects.

out around the time of the injection. I would be shaking, sweating, very anxious and on the verge of tears and had a sensation of impending doom.

When I was going through these periods I did not want to be left alone. I needed Colin's support until they passed which was usually a couple of days.

It was a good job I had been warned that there was a possibility that the treatment could make old symptoms re-appear. It certainly did have that effect plus some new problems. I had to carry a bottle of water everywhere I went, as I couldn't stop drinking, which in turn meant that if out I was always searching for a toilet.

At last I had found the reason for the weight gain and fluid. When I cut out all everyday foods around injection time the fluid vanished. My arms were particularly noticeable in that they went a lot thinner. The whole of my forearms had been very podgy and the skin taught, my watch was very tight as were my rings on my fingers. I had to stop wearing my rings.

My face had looked a completely different shape. It had become very rounded as if I was on drugs consequently my jaw line had disappeared.

There had been painful areas on either side of my nose below the sinuses. When touched these areas, as well as both sides of my neck, had felt like a sponge. At one time I had assumed that I had badly swollen glands.

Then I saw that the lumps on my shoulders had disappeared, my muscles didn't hurt any more nor did my joints. When I looked in the mirror I saw that my shape was more or less back to normal.

What a relief to know we had found the cause of more of my symptoms. The fluid was definitely caused by the

after one year of GPP almost normal portions of food + big change in energy but not sustained allergies.

After a year of the desensitising treatment I could eat almost normal sized portions of most foods.

There was also a big change in the amount of energy I had. So much so that at times there were flashes of the old me. I would be able to do a couple of hours gardening and still be able to make the lunch. There were some days when I hardly sat down.

It was these times which spurred me on to carry on delving to get to the reasons for the exhaustion. I really thought I was near the finishing post and started to plan ahead. What a big mistake that was.

As had been the case before I could not sustain this level of well being so I had to go back to living one day at a time.

We lost several hundred pounds having to cancel pre-booked holidays because my enthusiasm had overcome me. When the time came for the holiday I wasn't up to travelling. Never mind, my general level of fitness was far greater than at any time over the past several years and being able to eat normally after the rotation diet was superb. Now Colin and I ate the same meals again and life showed some semblance of normality.

My weight was not far off normal. I reckon I was only carrying about six pounds of fluid at that time.

Given my lack of recovery after following the coeliac diet, and that I had learned that a side effect of coeliac disease can be osteoporosis, I asked my G.P. if I could have a bone scan. This request was refused. I mentioned this to the nutritional doctor and he told me that a private firm, which used a different method of bone scanning, came to his premises periodically. This test involved scanning the bones in the ankles. My bone density was fine.

A year later I had an N.H.S. scan, because I saw another doctor, which showed that I had lost some bone density. I was amazed that this had occurred even though I was on H.R.T. I was advised, by the nutritional doctor, to add a combined calcium and magnesium pill to all the other supplements.

I had noticed that for most of the three years I had been on H.R.T. my breasts had been very painful. Since my mother had died from breast cancer aged sixty-two I thought that I had better discuss the issue with a new young G.P. I had been seeing. He advised that I should stop taking the H.R.T. immediately and never take it again.

> Stopped supplements because
> tingling - weak again. Started
> again + better afte two weeks.

CHAPTER 8

More new developments. For a couple of years the ball of my left foot had frequently been going numb and my toes had been tingling. I was not happy about this and mentioned it to the nutritional doctor. I asked if it could be a side effect of the pills but he didn't think so.

Nevertheless I stopped taking the pills for a few months because I was very worried. The numbness and tingling didn't improve and I went markedly weaker pretty quickly. Eventually I found that the cause of the numbness had been fluid. The tingling also disappeared but I do not know what caused that particular sensation.

All the old symptoms returned and the hair re-growth fell out. Nevertheless I didn't rush to restart the supplements just to make sure that stopping them was the reason for going down hill.

Because I waited for about three months by the time I did restart them I was not very strong at all, consequently it took weeks before there were any signs of improvement. This proved once again that the supplements were making a huge difference.

Two years later my need to drink had increased drastically and I was having to get up twice a night to drink a pint of water each time. Also my eyesight kept going blurred. It was suggested that I had better have a glucose tolerance test to see if I was diabetic. I was.

My sugar levels were not bad enough to warrant being put on insulin so the diabetes would be controlled by diet. Diabetics who take insulin can suffer from hypoglycaemia but not non-insulin dependant diabetics, so I have now been told by several doctors.

daily hypoglycaemic symptoms

Once again I did not conform to the norm as I was still experiencing hypoglycaemic symptoms on a daily basis.

Because of the combination of coeliac and diabetes I was advised to see yet another dietician. She said she couldn't help me, as she had never had such a complicated patient.

I must admit sometimes it is much better to try to work things out for yourself, as you know how you react, but once again I was facing a real challenge. Coeliac, diabetic and suffering from multiple allergies.

I was finding controlling my eating increasingly difficult. I started to think that my lack of energy was the effect of my blood sugar being too low because if I ate any form of carbohydrate I very quickly regained my energy levels.

I tried eating protein to see if that helped but there was no difference in my energy. The answer was to carry food in my pockets and I found that chocolate raisins or bananas were very good for keeping me going.

Keeping a check on my sugar levels was very important so I bought a testing kit of the type where a drop of blood is placed on a testing strip and inserted into a monitor. I was supposed to keep the level between 5 and 9 but invariably it would shoot up above 12 even though I had hardly eaten any carbohydrate. If I cut down further on carbohydrate I simply could not function for lack of energy.

The only way I could cope was to eat a fair amount of carbohydrate immediately before doing something and hope that the energy used would stop my sugar levels going too high.

Also I seemed to be having to eat far more protein than usual but noticed that as I got stronger this need disappeared. The only conclusion that I could think of was that I was not metabolising proteins, fats or carbohydrates properly.

Sometimes I forgot to take food out with me and I would invariably end up in a cafe eating a spoonful of sugar followed by something longer lasting like a piece of fruit. Within minutes I could feel the strength returning and off I would go.

Depending on how much I had eaten and how active I was, it might only be one hour before I needed to eat again. My energy levels dropped rapidly if I was doing something which required a lot of mental concentration, even faster than when doing anything physical.

Just prior to the glucose tolerance test I asked to have a thyroid test as we wondered if my thyroid was working properly.

We had read articles which said that some symptoms of an underactive thyroid are feeling very cold, dry hair and hair loss, nose and mouth twitching, lack of energy and low body temperature. I had all of those.

I had had an N.H.S. blood test several times over the years which had always indicated normal levels. We began to think the blood test might not be accurate.

One method of testing thyroid function is to monitor body temperature using a mercury thermometer. This is the test which was used years ago. Place the thermometer in the armpit immediately upon waking and before moving. Leave it in place for ten minutes and record the reading. Do this for a week. If the temperature if consistently below the normal temperature it could be as a result of an underactive thyroid. My temperature was very low. Would this explain why I always felt freezing cold right through in bed?

The private thyroid test involved collecting a 24 hour urine sample. We

> Urine thyroid test = low T3 + T4
> Tried adding copper, zinc + Selenium
> Very hard to treat T3 deficiency

were not at all surprised when it came back showing abnormal levels. The thyroid produces two hormones, T3 and T4. My results showed that I had too much T4 but was very low in T3. T3 is the active and most important hormone.

We thought it might be an idea to see an endocrinologist to see what he had to say. That was a very interesting meeting as he told us that most people are short of T4 not T3 and that it is very difficult to treat T3 deficiency. They normally only treat people with T3 deficiency who are brought in to hospital in a thyroid coma. <u>He thought it would be a good idea to try the nutritional approach which would be to take selenium, copper and zinc. More pills were added to my daily intake.</u>

Several months later the test was repeated and the results this time showed I was very low in T4 and T3. So far the nutritional approach had not corrected the thyroid function.

I decided to carry on with the selenium, copper and zinc and to forget any other form of treatment for the thyroid for the time being in the hopes that everything would sort itself out when we finally got to the bottom of all the deficiencies. The theory I was working on was that if I was treating too many things at the same time I wouldn't know exactly which treatment was working. One thing at a time would be better.

In the meantime yet more new problems arose. I thought my head had started tingling when I went near the microwave but didn't think anything of it for several weeks until the tingling became worse. Around this time I started to have a tight band around my forehead and numbness around my mouth. These symptoms also appeared if I went into the office when the computer was on.

My first thought was that it was something to do with the microwaves and the static so I had the microwave checked to see if it was leaking but it wasn't. Nevertheless I was not happy about using the old microwave so I bought a new one but this was no better. I tried to get something to cover the computer but there was only something to cover the screen.

The only way to resolve this was not to be in the rooms at all when the appliances were in use, because by this time the pain was excruciating within seconds of being in the room.

I also had pain when using the telephone. This did not please me at all as I still relied heavily on the 'phone for keeping in touch with friends. At first the pain was similar to mild earache then as the days went on it became much more intense until it too became excruciating and I could not use the 'phone at all.

One day I was having a telephone consultation with the nutritional doctor and explained that I had to use a hands free 'phone and the reason for this. I could manage a few minutes using this kind of 'phone before the pain was too much to bear. His response was "get yourself here now". We dropped everything and dashed of to see him. I was immediately put on an intravenous drip of magnesium.

About a year after I had started seeing the nutritional doctor I had a blood sample taken to test my magnesium status but this came back as normal. This test is not a reliable indication of what the magnesium levels are in the cells only the levels in the blood plasma.

The week after the drip I had a magnesium retention test. A healthy person would retain up to 20% and I retained 77%. The body only retains what it needs so I was clearly very deficient. The treatment was to be weekly injections in the buttocks, not the most pleasant experience as the pain builds up immediately after the injection, oral magnesium and soaking in a daily bath of magnesium salts for twenty minutes.

After following this regime for three months I had another retention test to see how much my levels had risen. They had come up 16%. There had been a very gradual difference in my energy levels but the most notable difference was that my sensitivity to the microwave, computer and 'phone had eased greatly.

This is a very exciting and fascinating phase of my treatment. Now I had to continue with the magnesium regime for several more months. Surely by the time my levels came up to normal that would be the finishing post.

Magnesium plays a big part in the working of many enzymes and I was sincerely hoping that it would help to *pain in calf muscles on incline*

sort out my sugar problems. Could this be the missing link?

When on holiday in Devon, several months previously, I was particularly strong so we went for some cliff top walks. The first day no problems. Absolutely super, just like the old days. The next day I experienced dreadful pains in my calf muscles when walking uphill. I thought this was connected to my blood sugar but it didn't go away when I ate.

The pains were nothing like the pain which can be experienced when muscles haven't been used for a long time.

There wasn't a problem when walking on the flat, only when going up an incline. The pain would build up until I couldn't bear it anymore. I would stop walking but the pain would continue to build up for what seemed like ages but was probably only several seconds, then it would subside, so off I went again.

Eventually I could only walk a few yards before this happened again and again. That was the end of the cliff top walks.

I had been hoping the magnesium would cure this problem but there wasn't any difference in this department.

It was suggested that I might have claudication. Something new to learn about.

This is narrowing of the arteries and is usually caused by smoking, something I have never done, but diabetes can also be a cause.

Off I went to see a consultant who decided it would be a good idea to have a test to see if I did have claudication. For the test I had to go to the Infirmary.

I was totally taken aback by the way I felt when we arrived in the car park. I did not want to get out of the car. When I started to walk towards the hospital I started to shake and cry, my heart was pounding, I felt sick and my legs were like jelly. I refused to walk any further. I kept looking down at the ground and did not want to see the building. I realized that I was having a panic attack.

I simply did not want to see any doctors. In the end Colin started to gently pull me along. Once I was in the hospital I calmed down.

The test involved monitoring the pulses in the feet and ankles prior to and after going on a treadmill. It was interesting that the pains in my calf muscles occurred when on the treadmill. The pulses in one leg were normal after the test, and only very slightly weaker in the other leg.

It was concluded that even though the pulses were good, as I had the pain and I described the symptoms as only occurring when going uphill, that I did have claudication as these were classic

> "claudatim" = water retention caused by allergies.

symptoms.

Initially when this possibility was raised I think I was in a state of total shock for several days. I could not believe that there was something else to contend with and felt exceedingly fed up. The answer is to stop the narrowing of the arteries getting any worse by limiting the amount of fat and sugar which is eaten. There is no cure.

When walking up an incline I discovered that if I slowed right down to a crawl when the pain started and I didn't try to go any faster I would eventually get to the top of the hill.

As usual, on reflection, I did not necessarily accept that I definitely had claudication. As my pulses were normal surely it could be possible that something else was causing the pain.

It was to be a year later when I worked out that the pain was caused by fluid retention in my calf muscles, a side effect of the allergies.

Sometimes the muscles would be very swollen and rock hard to the touch, and when pressed with a finger a white impression would be left. This is a sign of fluid retention.

CHAPTER 9

Although the Enzyme Potentiated Desensitisation had worked in that I had gradually with each successive treatment been able to lead a much better life, I did not like the fact that for four or five weeks after the injection I felt really knocked out with all the old feelings.

Also I was still finding the eating around treatment time, and the having to drink almost continuously, day and night, for weeks, horrendous.

It was interesting to note that I had developed some new symptoms since having E.P.D. Apparently this can happen. I had never experienced suicidal thoughts or such a feeling of impending doom before E.P.D. Colin and I found these episodes very disturbing.

I now had very prickly, sore eyes, spots, bloating, joints which would swell within minutes of eating, sometimes to such an extent that I couldn't bend my fingers.

I remember the times well when a finger joint would become bright red with inflammation, the skin very taught and excruciatingly painful to touch. As the pain gradually started to subside, usually within a couple of hours, I would try to gently massage the joint and was surprised to find that it felt granular, as though there were tiny crystals surrounding the joint. On occasions my toes would be affected similarly. The swelling normally subsided within two or three days.

All other joints tended to hurt and ache generally without any external evidence of inflammation. When I turned my neck or moved my shoulder joints I could hear a grating sound.

Earache was another new problem. Within minutes of eating I would have painful earache.

I took to wearing clothes with elasticated waists as my stomach would swell to such an extent, after eating certain foods, that I looked nine months pregnant.

Tiny clear spots appeared on the back of my hands in between the joints. Just the odd one to start with then as time went by more and more started to appear. They were very itchy and if scratched became very sore. Gradually they turned into scaly dry patches.

Eventually I realised that this was eczema. The culprits for causing this were black pepper, milk and capsicums, red and orange peppers.

E.P.D. is a very good method of desensitisation. However on reflection I think that as I was allergic to so many foods, coeliac and diabetic it was not surprising that I found it so difficult to cope, around treatment time, with the need to avoid foods which I was allergic to.

I started to wonder if I could go on with it.

I had heard of another method of desensitisation, neutralisation, and seriously considered changing to that. The only thing that was putting me off was that I would have to inject myself every day with the vaccine.

After dithering for months over what course to take in the end it was an easy decision because the last E.P.D. I had went wrong and sensitised instead of desensitised.

This was because I ate too much, not normal amounts but obviously enough to upset things, of some foods. I was in severe pain, because I had every symptom I had ever experienced all at the same time, and exceedingly fed up for several weeks. Once again I hardly slept. This was the last straw.

Certain foods were sending me to sleep. It was as if I had been drugged. Within minutes of eating a pear my eyes would start to close and I would have to go to sleep for a couple of hours. I could not fight it. Corn also had the same effect.

Rice had completely the opposite effect. I became hyperactive rushing round cleaning out drawers and cupboards, not something I'm normally known for, and unable to sit down. My heart was thudding and I couldn't concentrate. When the effect of the food wore off, whether it was sleeping or hyperactivity, I was left feeling totally drained usually for the rest of the day.

Once my mind was made up I asked the nutritional doctor to refer me to an allergy clinic which he sometimes referred patients to.

It was several weeks before I had an appointment at the clinic and by this time I had not been able to eat grains or potato at all for a couple of months. If I ate the tiniest amount of corn I would

Skin prick testing.
~~DESENSITISATION~~
NEUTRALISATION

suffer severe stomach upsets. As a result of these stomach upsets I lost half a stone which was weight I could ill afford to lose. To stop myself losing any more weight I lived off fruit, parsnips, beetroot and other vegetables for carbohydrate and the stomach upsets stopped. Eating this way I felt reasonably well but didn't have much energy and I was permanently freezing cold.

After a consultation with the consultant at the allergy clinic an appointment was made to start having skin prick testing to see exactly what I was allergic to. This involved having a dose of the allergen injected just under the surface of the skin then waiting for several minutes to see if there was a reaction.

As several tests have to be done for each food to find the correct neutralising dose I ended up with twenty nine pricks on my arm. All seven foods that were tested that day were positive and I was given a vaccine to take home so that I could start injecting myself immediately.

The second visit three foods were tested. Again all were positive and were added to the vaccine. I was told that it could take up to a month before results were seen but that some people see the benefit earlier than that.

I asked for the ingredients of the gluten free foods to be tested first, those are corn, rice, potato and soya, as I had not been able to eat any of them for ages due to the fact that they upset my stomach. It was particularly interesting to note that when potato was tested within a couple of minutes I needed to drink a lot of water.

All the foods made me feel an urgent need to sleep and also made me feel very weak. I was struggling to lift my arms. In fact I felt exactly as I had the two years I had been lying down.

Colin stayed some of the time the testing was being done and I'm glad that he did because he had been sceptical when, over the years, I had said that I thought that nearly every food I ate affected me. He found it absolutely fascinating when he saw the reactions I had to the testing.

We realised we were definitely on the right track. I felt vindicated.

I should have had this method of testing years ago. The blood tests were nowhere near as accurate.

Apparently, I was told, allergies can be the cause of needing to drink a lot and of hypoglycaemic symptoms.

The day following each test the pricks, except the ones which were related to the neutralising dose, on my arm had a swelling about the size of my thumb nail. My arm looked a horrendous mess, and was painful, as the swellings merged into one and covered a large area on my upper arm.

My drinking was excessive. I was waking at midnight, one thirty and three thirty to drink two or three mugs of water each time and to pass urine. I had tested my sugar levels and they were not high at any time throughout the day so that was not the cause.

Thank goodness it had been explained that allergies could cause terrible thirst or I would have been wondering what was going on.

My reactions to all foods were heightened and I also felt exceedingly tired but this improved gradually over several days. These aspects were similar to the reactions to E.P.D. but once all the testing had been done that would be the end of it.

Fifteen foods are tested initially and injected for a month to see if this form of treatment is successful. If it is other foods and chemicals are then tested and depending upon the reaction may be added to the injection.

The first testing session I had twenty nine needles in my arm, the next day I injected my stomach for the first time with the vaccine and had a magnesium injection in my buttock. I was beginning to realize what it must be like to be a pin cushion.

After nine weeks of injecting the vaccine daily I could tolerate corn, rice and potato in very small quantities every three days without feeling too horrendous. It was interesting to notice that there was a very fine line between the amount I could tolerate without symptoms and the amount which brought on the terrible thirst. The other foods in the vaccine could be eaten in a slightly larger amount.

I still rotated all the other foods, which had not been tested, on a four day cycle to maximise my quality of life.

After another consultation to find out if the treatment was working it was decided that more tests would be carried out for other foods and chemicals. I was particularly keen to have gas and perfume tested as I thought that I had a problem with these when I was in the caravan. Every time I tried to cook with the gas in the caravan I experienced a tightness across my chest and had to leave the cooking to Colin while I stood near the door or outside.

The perfume in the chemical used in the caravan toilet had a similar effect which was most inconvenient so we left the windows open all the time.

After all the testing had been completed it was determined that out of fifty four foods tested I was allergic to fifty of those foods. The two chemicals I had tested were both positive. All of these were now in my daily injection.

It has now been explained to me that with allergies it is a question of load on the body determining the level of fatigue. If only one or two foods present problems then a feeling of tiredness may be experienced. If many foods present problems then the total load on the body is so great that it cannot function normally anymore.

Each allergen is seen as an enemy and histamine is released. Eat several foods at a time which are seen as enemies and masses of histamine is whizzing round the body trying to see off the enemy creating a feeling exhaustion. The more that is explained to me the happier I become about the last eight years. It all makes such sense and I realize that it is no wonder that I could not function.

CHAPTER 10

The twitches and pains in my muscles were infrequent at this time but one day, after having walked more than usual, I noticed all power went out of my right thigh muscle again. It was exactly the same sensation as the day I was first struck down over eight years ago. I couldn't lift my leg and I felt absolutely exhausted.

This took me by surprise as I was still having weekly magnesium injections and had been much stronger since having them.

Another visit to the nutritional doctor was needed. Apparently potassium plays a part in muscle function and magnesium and potassium work together, so it was decided to carry out a red cell potassium test.

low Sodium Salt and potassium Supp + consultation after 2 weeks.

Although my G.P. had carried out several blood electrolyte tests which included potassium the results had always been within the normal range. These had not been red cell tests.

The results of the red cell test showed a marked deficiency in potassium in the cells which was too great to be made up by diet alone.

I bought some table salt which was low in sodium and high in potassium and was advised to take a potassium supplement for a couple of weeks and then to have another consultation. It is not advisable to take potassium without medical supervision as too much can cause heart problems. Too little can also cause the heart not to beat rhythmically so I wondered if lack of potassium had been the reason for my peculiar heart sensations.

One day after taking a dose of potassium my heart started to beat irregularly. I tried to stay calm but my first thought was obviously that I had taken too much but then I remembered that a few minutes beforehand I had eaten some nuts. When I've eaten nuts before I have had palpitations, so I came to the conclusion that they were more than likely the cause.

The following day I made sure that I did not eat anything around the time I took the potassium so that I could be sure it was not affecting my heart. It wasn't.

One really good day I thought I would like to go to the local public swimming pool for a swim with Colin. I set off to swim the length of the pool with confidence relishing the feel of the warm water and the weightlessness. By the time I had reached the other end I was pretty tired so I spent a long time sitting in the bubble section.

When I had recovered my strength I set off again and then suddenly without warning in the middle of the pool I

Sudden loss of strength in arms and legs in pool.

found that I could not think straight and could hardly move my arms or legs.

Colin saw that I was in difficulty. He pulled me to the side of the pool and helped me out. I sat on the edge of the pool like a rag doll, my head on my chest as I did not have the energy to hold it up.

The lifeguards came to see if they could be of assistance while Colin dashed off to the changing area and got me some glucose tablets. Within a few minutes of eating them I was able to have a shower and dress myself although it took several hours before I regained much strength.

A few weeks later we went for another swim and the same thing happened again.

Another day I felt really strong so I went for a stroll in the village. Once again I completely ran out of energy and found that I did not have any food in my pocket. I had to stagger into the chemists shop and flop on to a chair.

The assistants gave me Lucozade to drink and some glucose tablets to revive me. A man in the shop offered to take me home as the assistants had been unable to contact Colin to ask him to come and collect me because he was in the garden and couldn't hear the telephone.

Onlookers find it frightening when I am in a state of collapse but we are so used to it that it doesn t worry us at all. Doctors we had mentioned it to had no idea why this should be happening.

Even though I have been taking copious amounts of nutrients for three years I still have deficiencies. I had hoped that taking the potassium would be the answer but so far it hasn't been.

Chromium can help diabetic/hypoglycaemic symptoms so I take that regularly along with the multi-vitamins and minerals, fatty acids, calcium and magnesium pills, zinc and vitamin C.

In my case it is vitally important to keep taking all the pills because of the excessive drinking. It is more than likely that I am flushing out a large amount of the nutrients so if I did not take the pills I would be depleting the already low levels in my body.

CHAPTER 11

The effect of the magnesium injections was slow and gradual so it was some time before I noticed an improvement in my energy levels. After six months of weekly injections in the buttocks I was much stronger than before and I began to feel really happy.

When I had the last injection I left the doctor's surgery feeling elated and liberated. At last there would be no more doctors, nurses or needles.

Now Colin and I could really get on with living without having to plan our lives around medical appointments.

I was not completely back to normal strength but I was anticipating that I would be in several months time when the new neutralising treatment for the allergies had fully kicked in. All my allergy symptoms were getting less severe by the month.

The hypoglycaemic symptoms had been much less severe and I had not been suddenly running out of energy completely. I have been told that magnesium is essential for the body to store and utilise glucose efficiently in the muscles.

One awful day, three months after the last magnesium injection, I noticed that the microwave was starting to make my head tingle again and that my energy levels had dropped substantially.

Once again I had not noticed the changes until I was pretty weak. When it started to take me days to recover from slight exertion I had to admit that I was back to square one.

My sugar levels were noticeably harder to control, my allergic reactions were heightened greatly and I could not sleep. I suffered bowel disturbances which were far worse than usual.

In fact I felt pretty miserable and depressed. I was easily reduced to tears and felt I could not cope with this yo-yoing anymore.

Having sampled several weeks of being able to lead a near normal existence made the return to not being able to function seem particularly cruel.

It was time to ask for another magnesium retention test to see if my magnesium levels had plummeted. The test showed that they had. I was very pleased with this result as it meant that at least we knew the reason for the loss of energy.

I did not relish the thought of weekly injections again but if that was the answer then I did not have any choice. Something was going to have to be done, to stop the fluctuating between having good levels of energy and very poor levels of energy, to save my sanity.

I am not sure if it was worse to be weak all the time or to have good periods and then to keep experiencing the steep drop back down to the bad periods, and the long haul back.

We started to suspect that I may not be absorbing magnesium from my diet. This could be because one of the long term effects of the allergies is diarrhoea or because of malabsorption due to coeliac disease.

The nutritional doctor suggested that I have a new test, which the N.H.S. does not do, which involves taking a single cell and watching under a microscope to see if the cell absorbs calcium and magnesium. This test is only carried out at a private laboratory in London. As I was not strong enough to travel the blood sample was taken at the surgery and Colin took it to London on the train.

The results showed that my cells were absorbing calcium and

magnesium but that my magnesium levels were still low, even though at the time the blood sample was taken I had had ten consecutive weekly magnesium injections.

The conclusion was that the allergies were the culprits for the continuing low levels of magnesium. Therefore it was decided that I should continue with the weekly injections for several more months until the neutralising treatment for the allergies was having more effect.

SUMMARY

When, after the first couple of years of ill health and all the investigations, it became apparent that I was not getting better Colin and I made the decision that however long it took we would do our utmost to find the cause of my chronic fatigue.

We never suspected that the journey we embarked upon would take eight and a half years, and thousands of pounds, before we would be satisfied that we had really identified the root causes.

The many and varied symptoms of chronic fatigue mean that it is common for patients to be sent to see consultants from several different specialities. As I found this tends to result in having to endure undergoing numerous expensive and sometimes painful tests, all to no avail.

At times the stress of my unexplained ill health has been unbearable but the fact that this was exacerbated by members of the medical profession made it even harder to bear.

It is crucial to have self-belief and not to accept everything that doctors say if you do not agree with them. This is not easy, and can really grind you down, as most doctors do not like it if you disagree with them.

I found the easiest way of coping with this aspect was for Colin to always accompany me into the consultation room for moral support, and for me to come out of the consultation on occasions thinking "silly fool" about the doctor. On those occasions I would then complain to my friends to get it off my chest.

Another reason I liked Colin to accompany me during consultations was because I often became very worked up and found that I could not always remember exactly what the doctor had said.

It has also been a lonely time, just the two of us struggling to understand what was happening to my body and to make sense of whatever medical literature we could lay our hands on.

Strength of mind and determination is a must to cope with the worry and the knock backs. Only talking to and surrounding yourself with people who are sympathetic and understanding is also very important, as it is soul destroying to waste precious energy trying to convince sceptics.

After all this time I still cannot talk about my experiences to most members of the medical profession without starting to shake, feeling sick and crying. I do not know how long this doctor phobia will last but I have been left with a deep mistrust. I was self-confident before becoming ill but that self-confidence is yet to be regained.

Colin paid several visits to the local City Library to plough his way through medical textbooks in the hope of coming up with something relevant to my illness. As far as I can recall he did not have any success.

He also used the internet to seek inspiration, finding only a small amount of information. Nowhere did he find any comprehensive information, articles, or books which contained all the answers I needed for all my problems.

This is why I feel so strongly about setting my experiences down in writing. I hope that some of the information may be of some help to other sufferers of chronic fatigue or any of the many complications I experienced.

There were numerous articles in the British newspapers which implied that chronic fatigue was psychological. These articles made me feel really annoyed and only served to spur me on to prove that this was certainly not true in my case and I am sure in most cases.

A survey of published medical papers on chronic fatigue indicated that while British doctors concentrated their research on psychiatric causes, doctors in most other parts of the world were seeking physical causes.

Many people with chronic fatigue may be depressed, but that would not be at all surprising given that they are suffering long term ill health with debilitating effects, without much hope of help. The depression may be as a result of the ill health not its cause.

In my case it has gradually become obvious that I had multiple complications which were inter-related, consequently I was caught up in a vicious circle which has been very difficult to untangle.

Any one of my physical afflictions could have been individually responsible for debilitating fatigue. All of them together were too much for my body to be able to cope.

It is too easy to treat one of the symptoms and assume that will be all that is needed to regain full health. Unless each problem is sorted out full health will never be regained.

A holistic approach with proper testing is what is needed. It seems logical that the malfunction of my auto-immune system, thyroid, sugar control, digestion, motor muscles and joints did not all occur independently.

What appears to have caused my chronic fatigue is coeliac disease. It is a condition which can be asymptomatic so I may have been coeliac all my life without knowing it.

If I had been diagnosed coeliac much sooner all the other problems may not have set in or at least not got to such a drastic level. I find it very difficult to comprehend why G.P's do not test for coeliac disease along with any other blood tests when a patient complains of fatigue or exhaustion.

On the next page is a chart which I have drawn to show how I think all my problems were inter-related and stem from being coeliac. It also shows how if the key elements are sorted out then everything else corrects itself.

The cause of other sufferers chronic fatigue could be any one or a combination of problems.

If the word coeliac on the diagram is changed to stress, long term illness, bowel diseases or poor diet and the lines are drawn to malnutrition and allergies, it becomes very clear that the same pattern emerges.

Untreated coeliac disease causes damage to the intestines therefore essential nutrients are not absorbed thereby causing malnutrition.

- diabetes
- fatigue
- weakened immune response

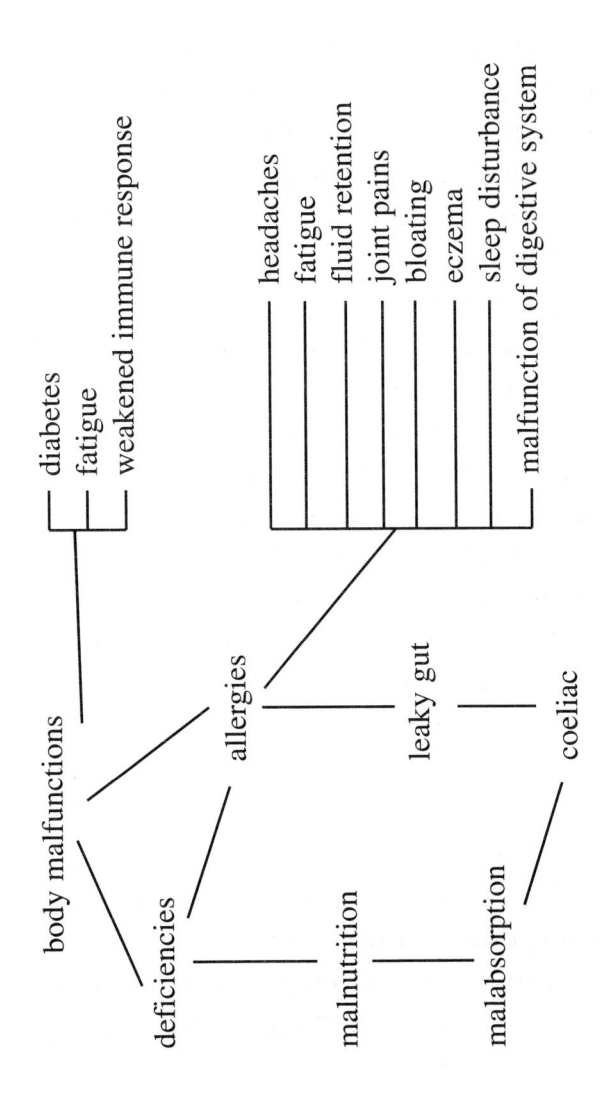

- headaches
- fatigue
- fluid retention
- joint pains
- bloating
- eczema
- sleep disturbance
- malfunction of digestive system

body malfunctions

allergies

leaky gut

coeliac

deficiencies

malnutrition

malabsorption

Damage to the intestines also resulted in my having a leaky gut which allowed tiny particles of undigested, or partly digested, food into the blood. This along with the nutritional deficiencies was the cause of the allergies.

The bio-chemical profile tests I had regularly after being diagnosed coeliac always showed that my electrolytes were within the normal range. These tests only showed the levels of chemicals in the blood plasma.

Blood plasma electrolytes do not reflect, in many cases, the level of the same element in the individual cells in the body. I now know that what was needed was to determine the levels in the cells. I was astounded to find that the levels in the plasma were normal but in some cases the cell levels were exceedingly low.

From talking to other coeliacs at the local society meetings and reading letters in the coeliac magazine I realize that late diagnosis and failure to regain full health is common. This should not be the case.

I heard of a young lady who had been anaemic and consequently very tired since she was a child. She had been taking iron supplements on and off for fifteen years. Only when she moved house and changed doctors was she diagnosed as coeliac. Once she cut out gluten from her diet she became stronger than she had ever been in her life. This is another clear case of not getting to the root cause of the problem early enough.

Coeliac Disease is incurable. Sticking rigidly to the gluten free diet is imperative so that the villi, the tiny protrusions in the intestines, remain their normal size, otherwise malabsorption will occur again.

Once malnourished nutritional supplements are needed to replenish the low levels of nutrients.

It has taken the whole of the eight and a half years for me to realize that one of the reasons I kept yo-yoing between being reasonably strong and being exhausted, was that the levels of nutrients in my body had not reached the optimum level.

As it was by doing too much before my nutrient levels were fully replenished I would deplete what reserves I had built up. If I had not taken supplements my levels would have remained very low.

Correcting the nutritional status is crucial for all bodily functions to work properly. Deficiencies can lead to a myriad of unexplained symptoms. The immune system will be weakened and this will lead to allergies.

Allergies in general can lead to nutritional deficiencies as they stop the body functioning properly. Amongst other symptoms they can upset the digestive system, causing diarrhoea, and therefore malabsorption.

Further complicating my search for the answer to my chronic fatigue was the fact that there was sometimes more than one problem causing the same symptoms.

Another cause of the yo-yoing was the allergic reactions. I could be out shopping with Colin one minute and hardly able to stand up or walk the next. Severe reactions to some foods came on suddenly, without any warning.

This made life exceedingly difficult. It was not unusual to have to find a chair in shops so that I could sit down before I collapsed on the floor. Once my body was on overload with reactions then it would be days of very careful eating before the reactions would pass.

Only by reading an article on allergies and recognising that the symptoms described fitted my symptoms did I start to explore this avenue. It had never occurred to me before that I might have allergies, let alone the extent of them.

It would have saved a lot of time if I had not bothered with the blood testing for the allergies but had had the skin prick testing in the first place. In my opinion this is the best test.

The reactions I experienced when being tested by the skin prick method were identical to the reactions when a food had been eaten, and the clear signs of large red weals on my arms meant that I now had indisputable evidence of multiple allergies. I knew then that I had found the cause of some of my problems.

Being allergic to so many foods and also chemicals I needed to have desensitising treatment. Most members of the medical profession regard this treatment as controversial but I knew that I could not go on without trying it.

I saw a doctor who had been practising nutritional and Enzyme Potentiated Desensitising treatment for twenty years, and went to a specialist allergy clinic which carried out the skin prick testing and the neutralising method of desensitisation. Both of these contacts had been by personal recommendation.

For two years I had Enzyme Potentiated Desensitisation but because I had complications, coeliac and diabetes, which made it hard for me to cope with this method, I decided to change to the neutralisation method of desensitisation. After a year on this treatment I am now able to eat most foods every two days without experiencing any bad reactions. Another few months and eating should be a lot easier again.

Once allergies have set in there will always be a susceptibility to them and I have been warned that I will have to be careful with my eating for the rest of my life.

Magnesium has been the final piece in the jigsaw. I am still having weekly injections but the difference in my energy levels is enormous. I can use the computer all day and use the microwave without any sign of pain, my sugar levels are much easier to control and I do not suffer stomach upsets. I can walk two miles easily now.

It is as though my whole body is starting to function normally again and everything is sorting itself out. Every week I feel stronger. Life is very nearly back to how it used to be eight and a half years ago.

I shall continue to take multi-vitamin and mineral supplements for the rest of my life as I clearly have a digestive system which is not functioning 100 per cent.

When I have finished having the weekly magnesium injections I may have to have occasional magnesium injections for the rest of my life to maintain the correct levels. That would be no problem at all.